Contents

What Is Whole 30 Diet?

The Whole 30 diet is a month-long elimination diet to support overall health. The central premise of the diet is that food you eat should make you healthier, but the creators of the program say that many common foods found in Western diets—including sugar, alcohol, grains, dairy, legumes, and certain food additives—can be harmful to your overall health, well-being, and energy levels.

The Whole 30 program was created in 2009 by sports nutritionists Melissa Hartwig Urban and Dallas Hartwig, who co-wrote the New York Times bestseller, "It Starts With Food." The co-founders have said that the diet was "born of science and experience." In practice, it is not a diet, but a short-term nutritional reset that claims to eliminate several food groups that could adversely affect the body, allowing the body to heal and repair itself.

During the 30 days, you eat whole, unprocessed foods, like fruits, vegetables, animal protein, nuts, and healthy fats. After 30 days, you slowly reintroduce off-limits food groups to check for reactions. The program is not a weight-loss plan, but many people find they lose weight on the Whole30 diet. Since the goal of the program is improved health, it is recommended that you don't weigh yourself or take body measurements for the 30 days.

In order for the Whole 30 diet to be effective, you must stick to the eating plan for the 30-day duration. This means that just one taste of any off-limits food can disrupt the healing cycle, according to the co-founders.

Proponents following the Whole 30 diet believe the plan can help:

- Heal the digestive tract

- Balance the immune system

- Eliminate food cravings

- Improve medical conditions

- Boost energy and metabolism

- Promote weight loss

- Change how you think about food

What You Need to Know

The program is based on research on how different nutrients can affect the body. Foods allowed on the plan must meet the diet's four so-called "Good Food" standards. On the Whole 30 diet, the food you eat should:

1. Promote a healthy psychological response

2. Promote a healthy hormonal response

3. Support a healthy gut

4. Support immune functions and minimize inflammation

The Whole 30 plan does not restrict the timing of meals, however, it recommends eating three meals a day and not snacking in between.

While the initial program lasts for 30 days, the reintroduction period can take time. During this period, it is recommended that you add one food group back in at a time, eating several servings of a variety of foods in the group over the course of three days while still remaining true to the rest of the Whole 30 plan.

Food groups can be added back in any order, however, some people choose to do legumes first, then non-gluten grains, followed by dairy, and then gluten-containing grains. In evaluating food upon reintroduction, it is important to pay attention to any symptoms, including gastric problems, rashes, body pain, or energy dips, that occur.

What Can You Eat?

When following the Whole 30 plan, you focus on eating whole, unprocessed foods including animal protein, vegetables, fruits, nuts, and healthy fats. At the same time, you avoid grains, legumes, dairy, added sugar, artificial sugar, alcohol, and certain additives.

The rules are simple but strict. Eat moderate portions of meat, seafood, and eggs; lots of vegetables; fruit; plenty of natural fats; and herbs, spices, and seasonings. Eat foods with very few, pronounceable ingredients or no ingredients because they're whole and unprocessed. Do not eat the foods to be avoided, even in small amounts, for 30 days.

After 30 days of following the Whole 30 eating plan, the off-limits foods are slowly reintroduced one at a time to see if anything triggers a reaction.

What to Eat

- Meat

- Poultry

- Seafood

- Eggs

- Vegetables

- Fruit

- Natural fats

- Nuts

- Vinegar (except for malt vinegar)

- Coconut aminos

- Herbs, spices, and seasonings

What Not to Eat

- Sugar and artificial sweeteners

- Alcohol

- Grains

- Legumes, including soy and peanuts

- Dairy

- Additives, including carrageenan, MSG, or sulfites

- Certain seed and vegetable oils

On the Whole 30 diet, all animal proteins (except dairy), vegetables, fruits, natural fats, most nuts, and most herbs, spices, and seasonings are allowed, which offers a lot more variety than what appears at first glance. The restrictions are clear-cut and require reading labels to ensure you don't inadvertently eat off-limit foods:

• No added sugar—real or artificial. This includes maple syrup, honey, agave nectar, coconut sugar, date syrup, stevia, Splenda, Equal, Nutrasweet, xylitol, and sugar alcohols. Small amounts of fruit juice used as a sweetener in recipes, however, is allowed, and whole fruits are not restricted.

• No alcohol. Do not drink alcoholic beverages or eat foods prepared with alcohol, even if it is cooked out.

• No grains. This includes wheat, rye, barley, oats, corn, rice, millet, bulgur, sorghum, sprouted grains, quinoa, amaranth, and buckwheat.

• Avoid most legumes. This includes beans of all kinds (black, red, pinto, navy, white, kidney, lima, fava, etc.), peas, chickpeas, lentils, peanuts, peanut butter, and soy and soy products (including soy sauce, miso, tofu, tempeh, edamame, and soy lecithin). Foods like green beans and sugar snap peas are not legumes and can be enjoyed on Whole 30.

• No dairy. This includes cow, goat, or sheep's milk products like milk, cream, cheese, kefir, yogurt, sour cream, ice cream, or frozen yogurt. The only exceptions are ghee and clarified butter, in which the milk proteins have been removed.

• Avoid certain seed and vegetable oils. This includes canola (rapeseed), chia, corn, cottonseed, flax (linseed), grapeseed, hemp, palm kernel, peanut, rice bran, safflower, sesame, soybean, and sunflower.

• No carrageenan, MSG, or sulfites. If these additives appear in any form on food labels, don't consume them.

• No baked goods, "junk foods," or treats with "unapproved" ingredients.

Sample Shopping List

The Whole 30 diet eliminates dairy, grains, legumes, sugar, artificial sweeteners, other additives, and alcohol for 30 days. The following shopping list offers suggestions for getting started on this plan. Note that this is not a definitive shopping list and you may find other foods that work better for you.

- Dark leafy greens (spinach, kale, Swiss chard, bok choy)

- Veggies (broccoli, cauliflower, Brussels sprouts, sweet potatoes, bell peppers, eggplant, carrots, cucumbers)

- Fruits (avocado, grapefruit, oranges, berries, bananas, apples)

- Lean animal protein sources (chicken breast, lean cuts of beef, pork tenderloin)

- Fresh or frozen fish (halibut, cod, salmon, snapper, sea bass, shrimp)

- Nuts (walnuts, almonds, cashews)

- Oils (olive oil, coconut oil)

- Organic non-dairy plant milk (carrageenan-free)

- Compliant seasonings (amino acids, malt vinegar, turmeric)

- Eggs

Pros and Cons

Pros

- Emphasizes wholesome, real food

- No weighing or measuring

- No fasting or complicated meal timing

- No essential special products or supplements to buy

- Coffee is allowed

Cons

- Very restrictive diet

- Meal planning and preparation required

- Difficult to follow in social settings

- No "wiggle room" for 30 days

- Must read food labels

The Whole30 Program isn't right for everyone, but those who have completed the program praise its effectiveness in improving energy, mental clarity, and overall wellness. Review the pros and cons before trying this eating plan.

Pros

Nutrient-Dense

The Whole 30 plan is filled with healthy, nutritionally dense whole foods, including protein, vegetables, fruits, and healthy fats. Most people report feeling better physically, mentally, and emotionally on this healthy-eating plan.

May Reveal Food Sensitivities

As an elimination diet, it allows you to identify foods that may trigger allergies or sensitivities. This is a clinical, time-honored approach and can work for the purpose of identifying trigger foods in order to minimize symptoms.

Restricts Added Sugar and Processed Foods

Nutrition experts also agree that removing added sugars and processed foods from our diet, like Whole 30 recommends, is a good thing. Reducing added sugar intake decreases inflammation, reduces illness, and improves overall health.

No Restriction on Compliant Foods

While several foods are not allowed during the Whole30 diet, there is no restriction on the amount of compliant foods allowed, meaning calories are not restricted and you can eat to fullness. The plan does not require fruits and vegetables to be organic or animal protein to be grass-fed or cage-free.

Cons

Very Restrictive

The Whole 30 plan eliminates several foods that are commonly found in the standard American diet and in most processed and pre-prepared foods.

Meal Planning Required

When following the Whole 30 diet plan, you need to carefully read food labels, avoid most restaurants and takeout, plan ahead, and prepare most of your meals from scratch. This can be time-consuming and many people find this to be the most challenging part of the plan.

Difficult to Socialize

The strict diet and no alcohol policy can make socializing difficult. Dining in restaurants and at other people's homes can be challenging. In addition, the program removes many foods that are physically addictive, like sugar and alcohol, and stopping these foods cold turkey could result in physical withdrawal symptoms. It is recommended to slowly wean yourself off sugar and alcohol prior to officially starting the 30-day plan.

Strict and Regimented

Because Whole 30 is an elimination diet, there is no deviation allowed for 30 days. Just one bite of an off-limit food can disrupt the healing cycle and require the clock to be reset back to day one, according to the diet's co-founders. Because the program was created by sports nutritionists with a tough-love coaching approach, some people may find it off-putting and insensitive instead of motivational.

Health Benefits

Doctors commonly prescribe elimination diets to patients with potential allergies, digestive problems, rashes, or difficult-to-diagnose symptoms. The Whole 30 eliminates some potentially problematic food groups for a month, then the foods are slowly reintroduced one at a time.

Most people who follow a Whole 30 diet discover some of these foods cause stomach upset, body aches, headaches, fatigue, rashes, or other uncomfortable symptoms upon reintroduction.

The main health benefits of an elimination diet plan like Whole 30 come from avoiding potentially unhealthy or problematic foods and identifying those to avoid long-term. The following is a summary of why certain foods may cause problems, according to peer-reviewed studies and additional research compiled in the Whole 30 co-founders' book, "It Starts With Food."

Added Sugar and Artificial Sweeteners

Few people would argue that sugar and artificial sweeteners are good for you. Foods with lots of added sugar are addictive and full of empty calories.

Artificial sweeteners mimic sugar and are linked to various health conditions including cancer, bowel disease, migraines, autoimmune disorders, and more. But studies investigating the link between these conditions and artificial sweeteners have yielded inconsistent results.

A research review published in the British Journal of Sports Medicine in 2018 confirms that sugar is addictive due to natural opioids released by sugar consumption.In addition, a 2017 review published in the journal Current Gastroenterology Reports found that artificial sweeteners contribute to metabolic syndrome and obesity by disrupting satiety signals, leading to increased calorie consumption.

Alcohol

Alcohol does not have any redeeming health benefits, according to the Whole 30 co-founders. It is a neurotoxin, addictive, and provides empty calories.

Alcohol also inhibits decision-making—so it's harder to stick to your diet—and interferes with hormones, glucose metabolism, and gut health. A 2015 study in the journal Appetite found moderate alcohol consumption before a meal increases calorie consumption by 11%.

Seed Oils

Some industrial seed and vegetable oils are high in omega-6 fatty acids, including sunflower, soybean, cottonseed, and corn oils, and are generally considered healthy. But a 2016 study published in Nutrients reports that the ratio of omega-6 to omega-3 fatty acids has increased from 1:1 to 20:1, leading to obesity, brain-gut problems, and systemic inflammation.

Minimizing omega-6 intake and increasing omega-3 consumption (as recommended during the Whole 30 diet) can help to balance out the ratio and is "important for health and in the prevention and management of obesity," the study authors conclude.

Grains

Grains make up a large portion of the American diet and the elimination of grains, as recommended in the Whole 30, sparks controversy with nutrition and medical experts. However, this is just a temporary elimination to give your body time to reset and determine if certain grains affect your health.

According to some research, grains can be problematic for some people for a number of reasons. They are easy to overconsume, promote inflammation, and the proteins found in grains—both in gluten and gluten-free grains—can be difficult to digest for many people. Grains are also calorie-dense.

For instance, a 2013 study in Nutrients found anti-nutrients in wheat and other cereal grains may contribute to chronic inflammation and autoimmune diseases. The study authors note eating grains can increase intestinal permeability and initiate a pro-inflammatory immune response.

Eliminating grains and eating more whole plant material is not necessarily harmful and may actually pack more nutrients for fewer calories. For example, replacing one cup of regular spaghetti with one cup of spaghetti squash saves 190 calories, boosts intake of vitamins A, C, and B6, and contains almost the same amount of fiber.

Legumes

Like grains, beans, peas, lentils, soy, and peanuts are often touted as healthy foods, but many people have problems digesting legumes. Legumes contain lectins and phytate, which may inhibit some of their nutrients from being absorbed during digestion.

In addition, soy contains phytoestrogens (plant-based estrogen) which can have a hormonal response in the body. Soy-based ingredients are very prevalent in processed foods, often found on labels as soybean oil, soy protein isolates, and soy lecithin.

While the Whole 30 co-founders admit the scientific case against legumes may not be strong, they recommend abstaining from legumes for 30 days and then deciding for yourself whether to include them in your diet once you reintroduce them.

Dairy

Despite milk's reputation as nature's perfect food—it has protein, carbohydrates, fat, and many nutrients—dairy products do not agree with everyone.

Milk contains the sugar lactose that many people lack an enzyme to digest (lactase, the active ingredient in Lactaid tablets), resulting in gas and bloating. Milk also contains the proteins casein and whey, to which some people react poorly.

Milk and dairy products can also contain hormones that may disrupt the endocrine system and lead to weight gain. According to a 2015 research review, certain hormones in dairy products may potentially provoke breast, prostate, and endometrial tumors.17

As with other foods prohibited on the plan, personal reactions vary. Taking a 30-day break from dairy products will give your body a chance to clear all the dairy from your system so you can determine if you are sensitive to it upon reintroduction.

Carrageenan

Carrageenan is a seaweed extract used to thicken processed foods. It's often found in almond milk, yogurt, deli meat, and other unsuspecting places.

A 2018 review published in the journal Food and Function reports that carrageenan may be linked to inflammation and digestive problems. In addition, its use as a food additive is on the rise, with increasing levels found in our diet. The study authors recommend additional research to determine if carrageenan may compromise human health and well-being.

MSG

Monosodium glutamate (MSG) is a flavor enhancer used in processed foods. The Food and Drug Administration (FDA) states that MSG is safe. And new research shows that not only is MSG safe, but swapping salt with MSG can help reduce sodium in your diet, which may improve overall health.19

However, scientists have also studied the effects of MSG as there have been reports of adverse reactions including headaches, rashes, hives, and nasal congestion. There have also been concerns about the link between MSG and other health conditions including low-grade inflammation and obesity.

While there is a large body of MSG research available, study results have been mixed and methodology is often called into question. For example, some studies may test quantities of MSG not typically consumed in the human diet. Authors of a large independent research review published in 2019 suggested that more high-quality studies are needed to fully understand the impact of MSG on human health.

MSG is hidden in foods under many names, including maltodextrin, modified food starch, hydrolyzed proteins, dried meat (i.e., dried beef), meat extract (i.e., pork extract), and poultry stock (i.e., chicken stock).

Added Sulfites

Sulfites are a byproduct of fermentation and occur naturally in many foods. They are also added to processed foods. People who are sensitive to sulfites can suffer from skin rashes, gastrointestinal problems, and cardio and pulmonary issues.

Health Risks

Though there are no common health risks associated with a Whole 30 diet, restricting healthy food groups can lead to nutrient deficiencies. Restrictive diets are also not recommended for those who've had or are at risk of developing an eating disorder since they can create an unhealthy obsession with food.

Sample Meal Plan

The Whole 30 plan advises three meals a day with no snacks in between. While Whole 30 cookbooks and the program's website provide recipes for Whole 30-approved meals, the following three-day meal plan offers additional suggestions for following the diet. Note that this plan is not all-inclusive, and if you choose to follow the Whole 30 diet there may be other meals that are more appropriate for your tastes, preferences, and budget.

Day 1

- Breakfast: 1 cup cooked oatmeal topped with 1/4 cup mixed berries and 1 ounce walnuts

- Lunch: 1 serving Low-Carb Salad With Chicken, Bacon, and Apple (use sugar-free bacon; substitute olive oil for Italian dressing)

- Dinner: 3 ounce serving Pistachio Crusted Salmon With Celery Root Potato Mash (3/4 cup mash)

Day 2

- Breakfast: 1 serving Omelette Roulade (omit feta); 1/2 grapefruit

- Lunch: 3/4 cup Avocado Chicken Salad (substitute cashew or almond yogurt for Greek yogurt) served over 3 ounces spring mix salad greens with olive oil

- Dinner: 1 serving Zesty Grilled Shrimp; 1 1/4 cup Roasted Rosemary Potatoes; 3/4 cup Roasted Beet Salad (omit feta)

Day 3

- Breakfast: 2 eggs scrambled or over easy; 1/2 an avocado; 8-ounce fruit smoothie

- Lunch: 1 cup cooked zucchini noodles topped with broccoli sautéed with garlic and lemon zest

- Dinner: 3-ounce serving grilled chicken breast served over 1 cup wilted kale; 1 cup Rainbow Vegetable Soup (omit green beans)

Whole 30 Diet Snacks

- Nuts and seeds with dried fruit

- Apple with almond butter

- "Pink Dream" collagen drink made with Vital Proteins Collagen Peptides, coconut milk, water, and muddled raspberries over ice

- Jerky

- Hard-boiled eggs

- 1/2 avocado sprinkled with sea salt and lime juice

- Roasted cashews with Everything Bagel Spice

WHOLE 30 DIET RECIPES

Trying new whole 30-friendly recipes is a great way to explore new flavors and find new favorite dishes while looking after your health. In this part are nourishing whole 30 diet recipes for you to enjoy.

EGG-FREE BREAKFAST BOWLS

Preparation time

45 minutes

Ingredients

• 3 sweet potatoes, cubed (whatever color you prefer)

• 6 tablespoons avocado oil, divided

• 1 teaspoon salt

• 1/2 teaspoon garlic powder

• 1 1/2 pounds breakfast sausage

• 2 heads of dino kale, roughly chopped and massaged

• 1/2 teaspoon salt

• 1/4 teaspoon cumin

• 1/4 teaspoon chili powder

- 1/8 teaspoon cayenne pepper

- juice of 1/2 lemon

- 1 cup pico de gallo*

- 1 cup guacamole*

- chopped cilantro, for garnish

Instructions

1. Preheat oven to 400 degrees F.

2. Line a baking sheet with parchment paper, toss sweet potatoes in 3 tablespoons of avocado oil and sprinkle with salt and garlic powder, then place evenly throughout the baking sheet.

3. Bake for 25-30 minutes, tossing them half way through to help brown on all sides.

4. Once the sweet potatoes have 15 minutes left to cook, place a large nonstick pan over medium heat and add the breakfast sausage.

5. Break into small pieces and cook until browned and no pink remains.

6. While the breakfast sausage is cooking, place another nonstick pan over medium heat and add 3 tablespoons of avocado oil to it.

7. Add the chopped kale and sauté for about 5 minutes, then add the salt, cumin, chili powder, and cayenne pepper.

8. Toss to coat and then add the lemon juice.

9. Once the potatoes are done cooking, build 4 bowlw – sweet potatoes on the bottom, then breakfast sausage, sautéed kale, pico de gallo,

guacamole, and top it all off with some chopped cilantro!

SWEET POTATO HASH WITH VITAL FARMS EGGS

Preparation time

1 hour

Ingredients

For the sweet potatoes

- 2 sweet potatoes, diced

- 3 tablespoons melted ghee

- 1 teaspoon salt

- 1 teaspoon garlic powder

- 1 teaspoon smoked paprika

- 1/2 teaspoon cumin

- 1/2 teaspoon chili powder

For the hash

- 2 tablespoons ghee

- 1 yellow onion, diced

- 1 red bell pepper, diced

- 1 yellow bell pepper, diced

- For the easy pico de gallo

- 2 tomatoes, diced

- handful of cilantro, roughly chopped

- juice of 1 lime

- pinch of salt

- Garnishes

- 4+ Vital Farms eggs

- avocado, thinly sliced

- cilantro, roughly chopped

- freshly cracked pink peppercorns

Instructions

1. Preheat oven to 400 degrees F.

2. Line a baking sheet with parchment paper and place diced sweet potatoes on top.

3. Pour ghee on top and sprinkle with spices then use hands to thoroughly toss.

4. Place in oven to bake for 25-30 minutes, until browned and soft.

5. While sweet potatoes cook, place a large cast iron skillet over medium heat.

6. Add ghee along with onion and bell peppers.

7. Sprinkle with a bit of salt then toss every couple minutes to help cook evenly until peppers are slightly golden – about 10-12 minutes.

8. While peppers are cooking, place all the mixture for the easy pico in a bowl, mix then place in a the fridge to chill until food is ready.

9. Once the sweet potatoes are done cooking, place them into the cast iron skillet with the

peppers and place over a medium-low heat to help held the flavors together and keep warm.

10. Lastly, place a large non-stick sauté pan over medium-low heat and grease to make sure the eggs don't stick.

11. Carefully crack 4 (or more) Vital Farms eggs into the pan and cook low and slow for about 5-6 minutes for over easy eggs with the white completely cooked through and yolks creamy and delicious.

12. When the eggs are done cooking, remove hash from heat then use a spatula to place each on top of the hash.

13. Garnish with freshly sliced avocado, a couple spoonfuls of pico, crack pink peppercorns, and cilantro!

BREAKFAST FRIES

Preparation time

1 hour 30 minutes

Ingredients

• 1/2 pound bacon

• 2 pounds yukon gold potatoes (or whatever white or sweet potato you prefer), cut into fry slices

• 2–3 tablespoons avocado oil

• hefty pinch of salt

• 1 pound breakfast sausage

- 4 eggs (or more depending on the number of people you are serving)

- 1/3 cup dairy-free cheese (I used Siete Foods Nacho Cheese Queso)

- 1/2 avocado, thinly sliced

- 1 tablespoon chopped fresh chives

- salt and pepper, to taste

Instructions

1. Preheat oven to 375 degrees F.

2. Line a baking sheet with aluminum foil then place a wire rack on top.

3. Spray wire rack with avocado oil spray, place pieces of bacon flat on the wire rack and place in

oven to bake for around 20 minutes, until slightly crispy.

4. Chop into pieces then set aside.

5. Leave oven on.

6. While the bacon cooks, cut potatoes into fry slices, toss in avocado oil, and sprinkle with salt.

7. Place in an air fryer without overcrowding the basket (I had to cook my potatoes in 3 batches) and cook at 390 degrees F for 15-18 minutes, tossing every 4-5 minutes, until potatoes are crispy.

8. While the potatoes are cooking, place a large nonstick sauté pan over medium heat, add breakfast sausage and break into small pieces, cooking until no pink remains, about 10 minutes.

9. Set aside.

10. In the hot pan with the remaining fat (about 2-3 tablespoons), turn the heat down to low, then crack 4 eggs into the pan to cook for 5-7 minutes, until whites are cooked through and yolks are still runny.

11. Heat up dairy-free cheese in a saucepan or in the microwave until warm.

12. To make sure everything is the same temperature, add the fries to the wire rack, top with the crumbled breakfast sausage, and bacon, and place in oven to bake for 5 minutes.

13. Top fries with eggs, dairy-free cheese, sliced avocado, chives, and sprinkle with a pinch of salt and pepper.

MEXICAN CHORIZO FRITTATA

Preparation time

Ingredients

- 1 pound chorizo

- 1/2 yellow onion, minced

- 2 garlic cloves, minced

- 10 eggs, whisked

- 2 (4 ounces) cans of mild diced green chiles

- hefty pinch of salt

- 1 beefsteak tomato, sliced into 4 slices

- 1/2 avocado, thinly sliced

- green onions, sliced, for garnish

- cilantro, diced, for garnish

- black pepper, for garnish

Instructions

1. Preheat oven to 350 degrees F.

2. Place an 8 inch seasoned cast iron skillet over medium heat.

3. Add chorizo and break into small pieces.

4. Once halfway cooked through, add onion and garlic.

5. Cook until brown and no pink remains.

6. Whisk together eggs, green chiles and salt.

7. With the cast iron skillet over medium heat still, pour the egg mixture on top of the chorizo then let the mixture cook for 10 minutes.

8. After 10 minutes, place tomato slices on top and put into the oven to cook for 30 minutes, until the middle is no longer jiggly.

9. Garnish with sliced avocado, green onions and cilantro and freshly cracked black pepper!

PIZZA EGG BITES

Preparation time

55 minutes

Ingredients

- 1/2 pound italian sausage

- 1/2 yellow onion, minced

- 2 garlic cloves, minced

- 1 cup pizza sauce

- 1 tablespoons chopped fresh basil

- salt and pepper, to taste

- 16–18 pepperoni slices

- 8 eggs

Instructions

1. Preheat oven to 350 degrees F.

2. Line 2 muffin tins with 16-18 silicone muffin liners and spray with coconut oil spray to make sure nothing sticks.

3. In a pan over medium heat, cook italian sausage with onion and garlic, breaking the sausage in to small pieces, until browned and cooked through.

4. Add italian sausage to a large bowl, add pizza sauce, basil, salt and pepper.

5. Mix to combined.

6. Then add 8 cracked eggs in to the bowl and mix to combined one last time.

7. Pour mixture into 16-18 cups leaving a little room in the muffin cup since the eggs will puff up while they cook.

8. Top each muffin cup with a pepperoni slice then place in the oven to bake for 30-35 minutes, until cooked through in the middle.

9. Then all you have to do is pack these guys in a sealed container and eat them throughout the week!

BACON & VEGGIE LOADED EGG CASSEROLE

Preparation time

1 hour 15 minutes

Ingredients

- 1 bundle asparagus, diced

- 8 ounces button mushrooms, sliced

- 1 red bell pepper, diced

- 1 yellow bell pepper, diced

- coconut oil spray

- 1/2 pound bacon

- 18 eggs, whisked

- 1 teaspoon garlic powder

- 1 teaspoon salt

- 1/2 teaspoon red pepper flakes

- 1/4 teaspoon black pepper

Instructions

1. Preheat oven to 400 degrees F.

2. Grease a 9×12 baking dish.

3. Place chopped vegetables on a baking sheet, lightly spray with coconut oil, then place bacon on top of vegetables, covering as many vegetables as possible.

4. Place in oven to bake for 30-35 minutes, until bacon is slightly crispy.

5. Turn oven down to 350 degrees F.

6. Remove bacon from baking sheet and chop into pieces.

7. Place bacon and vegetables in the greased dish.

8. In a large bowl, whisk together eggs, garlic powder, salt, red pepper flakes and black pepper until completely combined.

9. Then pour the egg mixture over the vegetables and bacon and mix to combined.

10. Place in oven to bake for 35-40 minutes, until the middle is cooked through and no longer jiggly.

LOX & CREAM CHEESE SHEET PAN BREAKFAST

Preparation time

1 hour 35 minutes

Ingredients

- 3 pounds yukon gold potatoes, cut in half

- 3 tablespoons high heat avocado oil

- salt, to taste

- garlic powder, to taste

- 1 bundle of asparagus, ends removed

- 1-2 tablespoons everything but the bagel seasonings

- 6 eggs

- 8–10 ounces smoked salmon

- 1/4 red onion, thinly sliced

- 3 tablespoons capers

- handful of fresh dill

- 4–8 ounces almond milk cream cheese

- coarse salt, for garnish

- black pepper, for garnish

Instructions

1. Preheat oven to 375 degrees F.

2. Place halved potatoes on a baking sheet and toss in avocado oil and sprinkle with salt and garlic powder.

3. Place in the oven to bake for 30-35 minutes.

4. After 30-35 minutes, when the potatoes are browned and slightly tender, use a potato masher to press each potato flat onto the baking sheet.

5. While the potatoes roast, place a small saucepan of water with a pinch of salt over high heat and bring to boil.

6. Once boiling, emerge the 6 eggs in the water and set a timer for 6 minutes.

7. Once they are done cooking, drain and add ice and cold water to the saucepan to let the eggs cool completely.

8. When the potatoes are done cooking, toss asparagus in a bit more of the oil then place throughout the baking sheet, in between the potatoes.

9. Top with the everything but the bagel seasoning then place into the oven for baking for another 15 minutes.

10. Peel the eggs then cut them in half and place throughout the sheet pan.

11. Then top the potatoes and asparagus with smoked salmon, red onion slices, capers, dill, dollops of cream cheese throughout, and coarse salt and pepper.

12. Serve immediately!

SUPREME PIZZA FRITTATA

Preparation time

Ingredients

- 1 pound hot italian sausage

- 12 eggs

- 1 cup pizza sauce

- 1/4 cup fresh basil, torn into small pieces

- pinch of salt

- pinch of black pepper

- red pepper flakes, to taste

- 1 green bell pepper, sliced

- 6 button mushrooms, sliced

- 6 pepperoni slices

- 2 cups arugula

- juice of 1/2 lemon

- 1 tablespoon olive oil

Instructions

1. Preheat oven to 350 degrees F.

2. Place a large cast iron skillet over medium heat.

3. Add sausage and use a wooden spoon to break into small pieces, until no pink remains.

4. Spread sausage evenly throughout the skillet.

5. Turn heat down to medium-low.

6. In a large bowl, whisk together eggs, basil, pizza sauce, salt, pepper, and red pepper flakes.

7. Pour mixture into skillet and let cook in the pan for 5 minutes.

8. Then top the frittata with green pepper slices, mushrooms and pepperoni.

9. Place in oven to bake at 20 minutes.

10. Toss arugula in lemon and olive oil and place on top of frittata before serving!

BARBACOA EGGS BENEDICT WITH CHIMICHURRI HOLLANDAISE

Preparation time

45 minutes

Ingredients

For the chimichurri (make the day before)

- 1 packed cup fresh cilantro

- 1 packed cup fresh parsley

- ½ cup olive oil

- ¼ medium white onion, minced

- juice of 1 lime (about 2 tablespoons)

- ½ teaspoon ground coriander

- ½ teaspoon ground cumin

- ½ teaspoon fine sea salt

For the pineapple jicama salsa (make the day before)

- 1/3 cup cubed pineapple

- 1/4 cup cubed jicama

- 1/2 jalapeno, minced

- 1/4 red onion, minced

- 1/4 cup cilantro, minced

- juice of 1 lime

- pinch of salt

- PaleOMG Barbacoa (put in crockpot overnight)

For the hollandaise

- 3 large egg yolks

- 1 tablespoon lemon juice

- ½ teaspoon fine sea salt

- dash of black pepper

- dash of paprika

- up to ½ cup melted butter or ghee

For the benedict

- 6 pieces of bacon

- 2 bundles of collard greens or rainbow kale (they will cook down a ton), roughly chopped

- salt, to taste

- garlic powder, to taste

- 6 eggs eggs

- cilantro

Instructions

1. For the chimichurri: place all the ingredients in a food processor or blender and puree until smooth.

2. Cover and place in fridge.

3. For the salsa: place all ingredients in a bowl and toss.

4. Cover and place in fridge.

5. Follow instructions for barbacoa.

6. Once barbacoa is done cooking, make the hollandaise: place the egg yolks, lemon juice, salt, pepper, and paprika in a blender and blend until well combined and smooth.

7. Turn the blender to medium-low speed.

8. Slowly pour in the melted butter and let the hollandaise thicken to your preferred consistency.

9. The less time you blend and the less butter you add, the thinner the hollandaise will be. If you prefer a thicker hollandaise, blend longer and keep adding melted butter.

10. Set aside.

11. Bring a large pot of water to boil.

12. Cook bacon over medium heat in a large pan until crispy.

13. Set aside.

14. Remove excess bacon fat, leaving behind 2 tablespoon in the pan.

15. Add collard greens and toss with salt and garlic powder.

16. Cook until soft and tender.

17. Lastly, to make the poaches eggs: Once pot is boiling, break each egg into a small cup, transfer it to a wire mesh strainer, swirl it around to get rid of the excess whites, and then return it to the cup.

18. Use a wooden spatula to swirl the water in a circle until the water is moving quickly.

19. Slowly ease each egg into the pot, spacing them evenly.

20. The eggs should continuously swirl and cook through, but feel free to continue to swirl the water a bit.

21. After about 2- 3 minutes, the whites should be fully set with the yolks still tender.

22. Use a slotted spoon to scoop out each poached egg.

23. Now to build the eggs benedict: place down greens, top with a piece of bacon cut in half, then add a hearty scoop of barbacoa on top along with a poached egg.

24. Mix about 2 tablespoons of chimichurri into the hollandaise then pour on top of the poached egg along with the salsa on top.

25. Garnish with a bit of cilantro!

SUPREME PIZZA FRITTATA

Preparation time

35 minutes

Ingredients

- 1 pound hot italian sausage

- 12 eggs

- 1 cup pizza sauce

- 1/4 cup fresh basil, torn into small pieces

- pinch of salt

- pinch of black pepper

- red pepper flakes, to taste

- 1 green bell pepper, sliced

- 6 button mushrooms, sliced

- 6 pepperoni slices

- 2 cups arugula

- juice of 1/2 lemon

- 1 tablespoon olive oil

Instructions

1. Preheat oven to 350 degrees F.

2. Place a large cast iron skillet over medium heat.

3. Add sausage and use a wooden spoon to break into small pieces, until no pink remains.

4. Spread sausage evenly throughout the skillet.

5. Turn heat down to medium-low.

6. In a large bowl, whisk together eggs, basil, pizza sauce, salt, pepper, and red pepper flakes.

7. Pour mixture into skillet and let cook in the pan for 5 minutes.

8. Then top the frittata with green pepper slices, mushrooms and pepperoni.

9. Place in oven to bake at 20 minutes.

10. Toss arugula in lemon and olive oil and place on top of frittata before serving!

5 INGREDIENT EGG-FREE SHASHUKA BREAKFAST BOWLS

Preparation time

50 minutes

Ingredients

- 2 sweet potatoes, diced

- 2 tablespoon ghee, melted

- pinch of salt

- 1 pound breakfast sausage

- 1 jar of Mina's Shakshuka Sauce

- 4 cups thinly sliced kale*

- just a little bit of salt

- green onions, for garnish

Instructions

1. Preheat oven to 400 degrees F.

2. Line a baking sheet with parchment paper.

3. Place diced sweet potatoes on the sheet then toss with melted ghee and a sprinkle of salt.

4. Place in oven to bake for about 30 minutes, until sweet potatoes are slightly crispy yet soft on the inside.

5. While sweet potatoes are cooking, place breakfast sausage in a large saute pan over medium heat.

6. Break up with a wood spatula into small pieces, until no pink remains and sausage becomes slightly crispy.

7. Then add the jar of shakshuka sauce along with kale and mix to combine.

8. Let simmer for about 10 minutes, until kale is soft and cooked through.

9. Sprinkle with a little bit of salt then mix.

10. Serve a scoop of sweet potatoes with a scoop of the breakfast sausage mixture on top and freshly sliced green onions for garnish!

SAUSAGE EGG CUPS

Preparation time

1 hour

Ingredients

- 2–3 chicken sausage, cooked and chopped

- 1 red bell pepper, chopped

- 1/4 yellow onion, chopped

- 8 eggs, whisked

- 2 garlic cloves, minced

- 1/4 teaspoon garlic powder

- 1/8 teaspoon red pepper flakes

- salt and pepper, to taste

- avocado, to garnish

Instructions

1. Preheat oven to 325 degrees.

2. Cook sausage until cooked through.

3. In a large bowl, add sausage, red bell pepper, yellow onion, eggs, garlic cloves, garlic powder, red pepper flakes, and salt and pepper.

4. Whisk until well combined.

5. Use a ladle to pour mixture into 8-10 muffin tins. (I used a silicone muffin tray and did not have to grease it. If you are using a regular metal pan, thoroughly grease all of it or use muffin liners.

6. Place in oven and bake for 35-40 minutes or until cooked through.

7. Garnish with avocado.

BREAKFAST PIZZA BAKED PEPPERS

Preparation time

1 hour

Ingredients

• 1 pound ground italian sausage

• 1 cup sliced mushrooms, chopped

• 4–5 basil leaves, torn

• 6 eggs, whisked

• salt and pepper, to taste

• 1/2 cup pizza sauce

• 3 bell peppers, cut in half, seeds removed

Instructions

1. Preheat oven to 325 degrees F.

2. Cut bell peppers in half and place in an greased 8×8 rimmed baking dish cut side up. (If any of the bell pepper halves are leaving to the side, ball up a piece of aluminum foil and place it in the crevices to help keep them sitting up right – this will keep the egg mixture for pouring out).

3. Place italian sausage in a medium pan over medium heat.

4. Break up with a wooden spoon. Once browned, add chopped mushrooms and cook until soft.

5. Lastly, add pizza sauce, basil and a bit of salt and pepper then mix to combine.

6. Whisk eggs in a large bowl then pour in italian sausage mixture and whisk to combine.

7. Use a ladle to pour mixture into each pepper half.

8. Place in oven to bake for 45-50 minutes, or until egg is completely cooked through and no jiggle remains.

9. Let cool slightly before eating!

EASY BREAKFAST CASSEROLE

Preparation time

1 hour

Ingredients

- 2 tablespoons fat of choice (coconut oil or butter or ghee, etc.), melted

- 1 large sweet potato or yam, diced

- 1/2 teaspoon fine sea salt

- 1 1/2 pound breakfast sausage

- 1/2 yellow onion, diced

- 2 cups chopped spinach

- 10 eggs, whisked

- 1/2 teaspoon salt

- 1/2 teaspoon garlic powder

Instructions

1. Preheat oven to 400 degrees.

2. Grease a 9×12 baking dish.

3. Toss diced sweet potatoes in fat and sprinkle with salt

4. Place sweet potatoes on baking sheet and bake for 20-25 minutes, until soft.

5. While sweet potatoes are cooking, place a large sauté pan over medium heat.

6. Add breakfast sausage and yellow onion.

7. Cook until no pink remains in meat.

8. Place meat mixture in baking dish, add sweet potatoes and spinach then add eggs along with salt and garlic powder and mix until well combine.

9. Place in oven and bake for 25-30 minutes, until eggs are set in the middle.

AIR FRYER ROTISSERIE CHICKEN

Preparation time

1 hour 10 minutes

Ingredients

- 1 whole chicken, about 3-4 lbs, insides removed

- 2 tablespoons ghee

- 1 tablespoon magic mushroom powder

- couple pinches of salt

Instructions

1. Remove insides from chicken and pat dry with a paper towel.

2. In a small bowl, mix together ghee and magic mushroom powder.

3. Pull back the skin on the breast side of the chicken and use a spoon to scoop some of the ghee mixture between the breast and skin and use your fingers to push the mixture throughout.

4. Do the same on the other breast until the ghee mixture is gone.

5. Sprinkle salt on the chicken throughout.

6. Pull out air fryer (I have the 6qt size) with wire basket inside.

7. Place the chicken breast side down onto the wire basket.

8. Close air fryer, turn the temperature up to 365 degrees F and time up to 30 minutes then press start.

9. Once the 30 minutes is up, use tongs or wooden spoons to turn the chicken over so the breast side is up.

10. Turn temperature back up to 365 degrees F and time up to 30 minutes then press start.

11. Once time is up, let chicken rest for 5-10 minutes before slicing!

MEDITERRANEAN CHICKEN SALAD

Preparation time

25 minutes

Ingredients

- 3 cups cubed cooked chicken, cooled

- 1 english cucumber, diced

- 1 red bell pepper, diced

- 1/4 red onion, diced

- 6 oz marinated artichoke hearts, drained and diced

- 1/3 cup kalamata olives, pitted and halved

- 3 tablespoons capers

- 1/2 cup avocado oil mayo

- juice of 1 lemon

- 3 tablespoons roughly chopped fresh dill

- 3 tablespoons roughly chopped fresh mint

- 1 1/2 teaspoon salt (or to taste)

- 1/2 teaspoon black pepper

Instructions

1. Place all ingredients in a large bowl.

2. Mix to combined.

3. Keep in the fridge to cool and help the flavors meld together!

4. Serve with almond flour crackers, plantain chips or in a gluten free roll.

5. Live your best life.

SHEET PAN SPANISH CHICKEN & POTATOES

Preparation time

1 hour 5 minutes

Ingredients

- ¼ cup ghee

- 1 teaspoon saffron

- 2 pounds of skin on, bone-in chicken thighs

- 1 pound chicken drumsticks

- 4–6 gold potatoes, quartered

- 1 bulb of garlic, cloves removed

- 2 teaspoons sweet paprika

- 2 teaspoons salt

- 1 teaspoon dried thyme

- 1 teaspoon dried oregano

- ½ teaspoon garlic powder

- ½ teaspoon onion powder

- ½ teaspoon fennel seed

- 3 leeks, greens removed, cleaned, and thinly sliced

- 3 chorizo sausages, sliced

- ¼ cup green olives, halved

- fresh parsley, for garnish

- fresh cilantro, for garnish

- lime wedges, for garnish

Instructions

1. Preheat oven to 425 degrees F.

2. In a small saucepan, heat up ghee and saffron for about 3-4 mintues, until the saffron becomes fragrant.

3. Place chicken thighs and drumsticks, potatoes and garlic cloves on a baking sheet.

4. Mix together all spices in a small bowl.

5. Using a basting brush, brush everything on the sheet pan with about half of the saffron ghee.

6. Then sprinkle half of the spice mixture on top of everything throughout the baking sheet.

7. Then place in the oven to bake for 20 minutes.

8. Turn oven down to 400 degrees F.

9. Add the leeks throughout along with the chorizo sausage.

10. Then brush the remaining saffron ghee on top of everything and sprinkle the rest of the spice mixture on top.

11. Place back in the oven to bake for 20-25 minutes, until chicken is an internal temperature

of 165 degrees F and the potoates are fork tender.

12. Top everything with green olives, chopped parsley and cilantro, and serve alongside lime wedges to squeeze on top before eating up!

CURRIED CHICKEN SALAD

Preparation time

15 minutes

Ingredients

- 1 rotisserie chicken, peeled, diced and cooled

- 1/2 cup avocado oil mayo*

- 4 stalks of celery, diced

- 1/4 cup raisins

- 1/4 cup cashews, roughly chopped

- 2 tablespoons curry powder

- 1/2 teaspoons salt

- 1/4 teaspoon turmeric

- 1/8 teaspoon cayenne pepper

- freshly cracked black pepper

- 3 green onions, diced

- cilantro to taste, roughly chopped

Instructions

1. Place all ingredients in a large bowl.

2. Mix to combined.

3. Keep in the fridge to cool and help the flavors meld together!

4. Serve with almond flour crackers, plantain chips or in a gluten free roll (this one is Against the Grain Gourmet)!

SLOW COOKER BUFFALO CHICKEN CHILI

Preparation time

8 hours

Ingredients

- 1 pound ground chicken

- 1 white sweet potato, peeled and diced

- 2 carrots, peeled and diced

- 2 stalks of celery, diced

- 1 yellow onion, diced

- 2 garlic cloves, minced

- 1 teaspoon chili powder

- 1 teaspoon smoked paprika

- 1 teaspoon cumin

- 1 teaspoon salt

- 1 cup tomato sauce

- 1 cup diced tomatoes (canned, not drained)

- 1/2 cup hot sauce (I used Frank's Red Hot Sauce)

- 1/2 cup broth (I used Epic's Beef Jalapeño Bone Broth)

- For garnish

- Tessemae's Creamy Ranch Dressing

- sliced fresno peppers

- sliced green onions

- fresh lime wedges (optional)

Instructions

1. This may get confusing, so good luck.

2. Place all ingredients in a crockpot (except for the garnishes) and mix together until combine.

(no, you do not need to brown the meat beforehand, no need to ask)

3. Cover and cook for 8 hours on low.

4. Once cooked through, mix once more to combine everything.

5. Garnish with Tessemae's Creamy Ranch Dressing, fresno peppers and green onions. A squeeze of fresh lime juice makes it even more fresh tasting!

FAJITA CHICKEN SALAD

Preparation time

55 minutes

Ingredients

- 2 tablespoons ghee

- 1 red bell pepper, diced

- 1 yellow bell pepper, diced

- 1/2 yellow onion, diced

- 2 garlic cloves, minced

- 1 jalapeño, minced

- 1 (8 ounce) can roasted mild green chiles

- pinch of salt and pepper

- 2 1/2 cup diced cooked chicken, cooled (I used a rotisserie chicken)

- 1 1/2 tablespoons fajita seasonings

- 1/2 cup avocado mayo

- juice of 1/2 lime

- 1/2 cup cilantro, roughly chopped

Instructions

1. Place ghee in a large saute pan over medium heat.

2. Once hot, add peppers and onion.

3. Cook for about 10 minutes, until the veggies begin to brown.

4. Then add garlic, jalapeño, and green chiles.

5. Sprinkle with salt and pepper and cook for another 3-4 minutes.

6. Add chicken and fajita seasonings to the pan and cook for another 3 minutes, until the veggies and chicken are coated in the spices.

7. Remove from heat and place in the fridge to cool for 30 minutes or until completely cool.

8. Mix the chicken and veggies with mayo, lime juice and cilantro then place in the fridge to cool for 1 hour and 30 minutes before eating!

BUFFALO CHICKEN SOUP

Preparation time

1 hour

Ingredients

- 2 tablespoons ghee

- 1 cup diced carrots

- 1 cup diced celery

- 1/2 white onion, minced

- 3 garlic cloves, minced

- 4 cups cauliflower florets (I used a frozen bag of cauliflower that was defrosted – it cooks quicker and a little better)

- 32 ounces chicken bone broth

- 2/3 cup Frank's Red Hot Sauce (less if you don't like it as spicy)

- salt and pepper, to taste

- 1 rotisserie chicken, pulled and shredded

- fresh cilantro, for garnish

- chopped green onions, for garnish

- Primal Kitchen Avocado Oil Ranch, for garnish

Instructions

1. Place ghee in the basin of the instant pot then press the sauté button.

2. Once the ghee begins to melt, add the carrots, celery, onion and garlic and sauté for

about 5 minutes, until onion becomes translucent.

3. Press the keep warm/cancel button, add the cauliflower, chicken broth, hot sauce and a hefty pinch of both salt and pepper, then secure the lid, close off the pressure valve and press the Soup button.

4. This will cook for 30 minutes once it comes up to pressure.

5. Once the soup is done cooking, you can let it naturally release or do a quick release.

6. Once you remove the lid, use an immersion blender to blend the soup until completely smooth.

7. Taste to see if the soup needs any extra salt or pepper.

8. Turn the soup back onto the Saute function and add the rotisserie chicken and let cook down for 8-10 minutes, stirring every 2 minutes to keep from sticking.

9. Press the keep warm/cancel button before serving.

10. Garnish soup with a swirl of ranch, hot sauce, green onions and cilantro.

JALAPEÑO POPPER CHICKEN SALAD

Preparation time

35 minutes

Ingredients

- 3 cups diced cooked chicken, chilled

- 1/2 pound bacon, diced and cooked until crispy

- 3 jalapeños, roasted

- 1/2 red onion, minced

- 1/2 cup Primal Kitchen avocado mayo

- 2 tablespoons hot sauce

- 1/2 teaspoon garlic powder

- 1/2 – 1 teaspoon salt

- black pepper, to taste

- chopped chives

Instructions

1. Dice chicken and place in the fridge to chill.

2. Cook diced bacon in a medium pan until crispy.

3. Remove and set on a paper towel to absorb the excess fat.

4. Place jalapeños on a the stove top over a high flame and rotate every couple minutes until the jalapeño begins to blacken and blister.

5. Once roasted on all sides and slightly softened, rinse under cold water and remove the blackened skin, then mince the jalapeño. (for less spicy, remove the seeds before slicing)

6. Add the chicken, bacon, jalapeño, red onion, mayo, hot sauce, garlic powder, salt, black

pepper and chopped chives to a large bowl and mix until completely combined.

7. Serve in lettuce wraps or on any gluten free or paleo bread you prefer!

CHICKEN BACON RANCH CASSEROLE (VIDEO!)

Preparation time

1 hour 5 minutes

Ingredients

- 1 medium spaghetti squash (about 2 1/2 pounds), cut in half

- 1/2 pound bacon, cubed

- 1 red bell pepper, diced

- 1 yellow bell pepper, diced

- 1/2 yellow onion, minced

- 2 garlic cloves, minced

- 1 pound ground chicken

- 1 teaspoon garlic powder

- 1/2 teaspoon salt

- 1/2 teaspoon black pepper

- 1/4 teaspoon cayenne pepper

- 1 cup Primal Kitchen Ranch

- 3 eggs

- chopped chives, to garnish

Instructions

1. Preheat the oven to 400 degrees F.

2. Cut the spaghetti squash in half lengthwise.

3. Place the squash cut side down on a baking sheet and bake for 30 to 35 minutes or until the skin gives when you press your finger to it.

4. Remove the squash from the oven and reduce the oven temperature to 350 degrees F.

5. Grease an 8×8 glass baking dish.

6. While the spaghetti squash cooks, place a large saute pan over medium heat, add bacon, and cook until crispy, about 10 minutes.

7. Remove and set aside. You'll want to leave behind about 2 tablespoons worth of bacon fat to feel free to remove any excess once bacon has cooked.

8. Add peppers, onion and garlic cloves and cook for about 10 minutes, until onion is translucent.

9. To the pan with the peppers and onion, add the ground chicken along with the garlic powder, salt, black pepper, and cayenne pepper.

10. Use a wooden spoon to break apart the chicken and cook until no pink remains, about 10 minutes.

BURGER BOWLS

Preparation time

50 minutes

Ingredients

- 4 yukon gold potatoes, cubed

- 3 tablespoons Primal Kitchen High Heat Avocado Oil

- 1 teaspoon salt

- 4 strips of bacon

- 1 1/2 pound ground beef

- 1 tablespoon Primal Palate Meat & Potato Seasonings

- 1/4 cup Primal Kitchen Garlic Aioli

- 2 tablespoon coconut milk

- pinch of salt

- 1 head of butter lettuce

- 1 large heirloom tomato, cut into 4 slices

- 1/4 red onion, thinly sliced

- 1 cup dill pickle chips

Instructions

1. Cube potatoes in small pieces. You want these pieces to be small and cubed evenly to help with

reducing cooking time and evenly cooking throughout.

2. In a bowl, toss potatoes in Primal Kitchen High Heat Avocado Oil and then add salt, and toss.

3. Place potatoes inside wire basket of air fryer and spread evenly throughout.

4. Close air fryer then turn temperature on air fryer up to 400 degrees and time up to 25 minutes and press start.

5. Keep an eye on the time because you will want to pause the air fryer every 5 minutes and toss the potatoes to make sure they cook evenly throughout.

6. Once finished cooking, sprinkle with a little extra salt on top while still hot.

7. While the potatoes cook, place bacon in a large nonstick skillet over medium heat and cook for 5 minutes per side, until crispy.

8. Set aside on a paper towel.

9. In a large bowl, use your hands to mix together the ground beef with meat & potato seasonings until combined.

10. Pour into 4 large patties and pat them down to make them pretty flat.

11. Add burger patties to the pan and cook for 5-6 minutes per side, depending on the thickness and how you like your burgers.

12. While the burgers cook, in a small bowl mix together garlic aioli, coconut milk, and salt until combined.

13. Once the burgers are done cooking, build the bowls – butter lettuce on the bottom, then a slice of heirloon tomato, burger patty topped with garlic crema, a few slices of red onion, some dill pickle chips, and a big of plop of crispy potatoes. Eat up!

INSTANT POT TACO STUFFED POTATOES

Preparation time

1 hour

Ingredients

• 3 russet potatoes, poked with holes throughout

- 1 cup water

- 4 tablespoons melted ghee, divided

- salt, to taste

- 1 red bell pepper, diced

- 1 yellow bell pepper, diced

- 1/2 yellow onion, diced

- 2 garlic cloves, minced

- 1/2 jalapeno, diced

- 1 pound grass-fed ground beef

- juice of 1/2 lime

- 2 tablespoons hot sauce (I used Frank's Hot Sauce)

- 2 tablespoons taco seasoning

- For garnish

- cilantro

- diced fresno peppers

Instructions

1. Preheat oven to 450 degrees F.

2. Wash potatoes and poke holes throughout.

3. Place water in the basin of the instant pot then place a steamer basket or wire rack inside and potatoes within.

4. Press the keep warm/cancel button then secure the lid, close off the pressure valve and press manual to high pressure and press the up button until the time hits 20 minutes.

5. The instant pot will have to come to pressure then the time will begin.

6. Once the time is up, let the pressure naturally release for 10 minutes then release any leftover pressure before removing lid.

7. Carefully remove the potatoes from instant pot using a towel or tong (so you don't burn yourself) making sure you don't break the skin, then use a brush to brush each potatoes with melted ghee and sprinkle with salt.

8. Place in oven on rack to crisp up. (You should be able to cook the potato in the oven the entire time it takes you to finish the taco meat, but keep an eye on it to make sure the potatoes don't burn!)

9. Discard water from basin and place back in the instant pot.

10. Press Sauté function and add 2 tablespoons ghee along with the bell peppers, onion and a bit of salt.

11. Sauté for about 5 minutes then add garlic, jalapeño, and ground beef and break beef into smaller pieces.

12. After meat has browned, about 5 minutes, add lime, hot sauce, and taco seasonings.

13. Mix to combine completely.

14. Press cancel, secure lid, close off pressure valve then press manual to high pressure and press the up button until the time hits 10 minutes.

15. Once time is up, quick release the pressure, remove lid and taste to see if the taco meat needs any salt.

16. Remove potatoes from oven, cut each down the middle, pour taco meat inside and top with cilantro and fresno peppers.

SLOW COOKER POT ROAST WITH EASY GRAVY

Preparation time

8 hours 30 minutes

Ingredients

- 2 tablespoons ghee

- 4 pound chuck roast, tied around the outside with twine

- himalayan sea salt, to taste

- 3 medium carrots, peeled and sliced

- 3 medium parsnips, peeled and sliced

- 1 medium yellow onion, cut into quarters

- 3 garlic cloves, sliced

- 1 tablespoon chopped fresh thyme + extra sprigs

- pinch of black pepper

- 2 bay leaves

- 2 cups beef broth

- 1/3 cup red wine (optional)

- 1 tablespoon honey

- 1/4 cup tapioca or arrowroot flour

- 1 batch of Cauliflower Puree on page 202 in Juli Bauer's Paleo Cookbook

Instructions

1. Place a large cast iron skillet over medium heat.

2. Once hot, add ghee.

3. Sprinkle salt on chuck roast then sear on all sides, about 2-3 minutes per side.

4. Place in slow cooker and put sliced carrots, parsnips and onion around the roast.

5. Top the roast with garlic cloves, a bit more salt, thyme and thyme sprigs and black pepper.

6. Put the bay leaves in the pot then pour in the beef broth and red wine.

7. Cover and let cook for 8 hours on low.

8. Once roast is done cooking, remove roast and place in a baking dish then use a slotted spoon to remove all the veggies and set in the baking dish with roast.

9. Cover with foil to keep warm while you finish the dish.

10. If you are making cauliflower puree, make it now.

11. For the gravy: Dispose of bay leaves and thyme sprigs from slow cooker then use an immersion blender to puree broth in the bottom of the slow cooker.

12. Once pureed, pour mixture into a large sauté pan and place it over medium heat.

13. Add honey and whisk.

14. Then while continuously mixing, add arrowroot or tapioca flour to the mixture, one teaspoon at a time.

15. Be sure to continuously whisk because it can clump up. Once all flour is combined and gravy has thickened, pour mixture through a mesh strainer to get rid of any clumps.

16. To serve pot roast: place cauliflower puree in a bowl along with veggies, pot roast that has been pulled apart with fork, and gravy on top!